Ahhh...
Feel & Look Human Again!
with Ergonomics and Skin Care

Ahhh...
Feel & Look Human Again!
with Ergonomics and Skin Care

Susan Kelso

Illustrations by John & Mike Serpentelli

Tate Publishing & *Enterprises*

Ahhh...Feel and Look Human Again!

Published by Tate Publishing & Enterprises, LLC
127 E. Trade Center Terrace | Mustang, Oklahoma 73064 USA
1.888.361.9473 | www.tatepublishing.com

Tate Publishing is committed to excellence in the publishing industry. The company reflects the philosophy established by the founders, based on Psalm 68:11,
"The Lord gave the word and great was the company of those who published it."

Cover and Interior design by Chris Webb

Published in the United States of America

ISBN: 978-1-61663-632-6
1. Health & Fitness / General
10.09.27

Disclaimer

The intent of our book is to share information for the health and well being of your body and skin.

Contact your *Physician* and/or *Healthcare Practitioner* with regards to any lifestyle suggestions within this book, *if* necessary.

The author, illustrator, and any other persons involved with this book assume *no liability* whatsoever for any persons, adult or child, due to or as a result of, the information herein.

Donations

10 % sales will support a 501C 3
Non-Profit Organization

Save our Strays/Rescata los Gatos, Inc.

Rescue to reduce the over-population
of homeless animals

www.saveourstrayssos.com

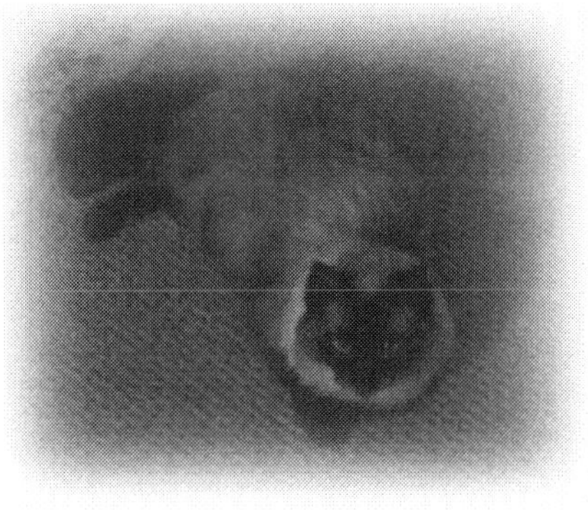

In Memory of Romeo, I Love You!

God has given each of us a gift. Use it to help each other…

1 Peter 4:10 (NLV)

Dedication

I dedicate our book to everyone that I have *touched* with massage therapy and skin care as you have been my inspiration and a blessing!

My belief is that we are all students and teachers, and it is our responsibility to teach what we learn with others!

Such simple, effective, and easy-to-do tips have been shared with family, friends, clients, as well as professionals, and now it is my pleasure to share them with all of you!

Acknowledgments

Special thanks to John and Mike Serpentelli
for their brilliance with my vision.

Many thanks to Anja, Doris, Ana, Gia, Susan,
Hanne, Maritza, Silvia, Mark, Abel, Yoan and others
for sharing their insights, expertise, and humor.

Heartfelt thanks to my family for
all of their love and support.

Much appreciation to everyone as I could
not have done this without *all* of you!

Mostly, I thank *God* for all of *His* blessings!

Table of Contents

Foreword

Hmmm … Human Habits and Skin Care

Humorous illustrations and simple explanations teach you how to take care of your body and skin with comfort and ease for your overall health, well-being and a more youthful appearance!

Your body has it's own *natural* design -

Do it, and life is good!

Do it *differently*, and you will feel pain and discomfort sooner or later!

Simple lifestyle changes give meaningful results!

My greatest desire is that when you read our book, you will be awakened and hopeful, and…

Ahhh… Feel & Look Human Again!

Preface

Wherever you go there you are, so take care of you, as it is the only place you have to live!

Since your pain and discomfort as well as premature aging are due to habit, injury, surgery, illness or genetics, it is often a surprise to most that the *root cause* is usually just a *habit!*

Your *often-known* or *unknown* lifestyle habits such as too much stress as well as poor posture and diet are due to both *preventable* and *unpreventable* causes.

Once you understand the *root causes* of your problems, it is so easy to make some simple lifestyle changes and…

Ahhh… Feel & Look Human Again!

Where stress starts, tight muscles and premature facial wrinkles follow!

Where tight muscles and premature facial wrinkles start, stress follows!

Introduction

Just a thought: *stressed* spelled backwards is *desserts*!

Simplify, simplify, simplify — stress is a *root cause* of disease and dis-ease as it affects your body and skin, as well as your mind and emotions!

Contrary to popular belief, your tight muscles and premature facial wrinkles are not *only* stress, and the *good* news is that you do not have it live with it forever!

Usually, it only takes up to a *few* weeks to form a new habit!

Once you begin to change a *lifestyle* habit, *encouragement* follows with *relief* and *renewal* as you feel and look better *sooner* rather than later!

Ergonomics for Proper Posture teaches you awareness of your *preventable* and *unpreventable* causes as well as how to change your *often-known* or *unknown* lifestyle habits!

Many of these common-sense tips you may already *know*, perhaps have simply *forgotten*, or may be *unknown* to you until now!

Ergonomics for Proper Posture

- Stress is not the *only* cause of your tight muscles!
- Your tight muscles are the *symptoms* and not the problem!
- The problem is the *root cause(s)* of your pain and discomfort!

Often the *root causes* of your tight muscles are just poor posture and lack of or improper support.

Surprisingly, these problems are easily *preventable* with some simple lifestyle changes such as *ergonomics* and *proper* support.

The answer is not to treat your symptoms *only* as it usually just masks the problem, may be ineffective, and cause possible side effects.

The *real* answer is to always treat the *root cause(s)* for relief and results.

Overall your tight muscles are *unhealthy* as they create stress, weaken your immune system, cause toxic congestion, possible injury, and zap your energy, just to name a few!

What are *you* doing to create your symptoms?

Usually, it is your *often-known or unknown* lifestyle habits, *especially* for a length of time at *work*, *school*, *play* or *rest*!

....

Since your pain and discomfort is usually *more* on *one* side of your body than the other, most often it is due to *lack* of ergonomics, and *unnatural* sleep habits.

Imagine yourself, or better yet, actually *do* some *unnatural* positions with your body, such as turning your head to *one* side while on the phone, computer, or sleeping on your stomach.

You will feel tight muscles with your back, neck and shoulders, and *more* on the side you turn towards only.

Stress will intensify your tight muscles, but it is *not* the *root cause* alone.

**If* it were *only* stress, you would feel the *same* tight muscles on *both* sides of your body, and not *more* on just one side.

....

Some *problem* areas and usual *root causes* due to *unnatural* positions, *especially* for a length of time

Upper Back, Neck and Shoulders

- lack of or improper support
- head turn or tilt
- head up or down
- stomach-sleep

Scapula(s)

- raise shoulder(s) up
- stomach-sleep

Lower Back

- lack of or improper support
- leg crosses
- raise arm(s) above shoulders or outward
- uneven leg lengths
- stomach-sleep

Legs and Feet

- lack of or improper arch support
- uneven leg lengths

Arms and Hands

- lack of or improper support
- raise arm(s) above shoulders or outward
- arm(s) and wrist bends
- elbow(s) leans
- hand(s) closed as in a fist

*Any *unnatural* positions causes tight muscles *sooner* rather than later!

Although exercise and relaxation give you *temporary* relief, it is simply *not* enough to undue the *many* hours of poor posture and lack of support.

Once you go back to your *often-known or unknown* lifestyle habits, you create the *same* tight muscles *sooner* rather than later!

Some lifestyle changes, such as *Ergonomics for Proper Posture*, help you be part of the solution and...

Ahhh... Feel & Look Human Again!

Some *preventable* and *unpreventable* usual *root causes* of tight muscles, *especially* for a length of time

- poor posture and diet
- lack of or improper support
- dehydration and deficiency
- hormonal imbalance
- overabundance of stress and fatigue
- lack of sleep and exercise
- sleep habits such as stomach-sleeping
- congestion of toxins and lack of oxygen

- inflammation or structural
- injury or surgery
- illness or genetics
- disability
- pregnancy and child care
- elderly and natural aging
- occupational

- negative emotions –
- anger and resentment refers to back, neck and shoulders - forgive and let go
- anxiety refers to stomach – live in the present
- fear refers to kidneys (lower back) - surrender
- grief refers to lungs – four stages are necessary -
- denial, sadness, anger and acceptance

*Negative emotions prematurely age your body

The good news for both *preventable* and *unpreventable* causes is that your pain and discomfort can lessen or even disappear once you stop the *root causes(s)*!

For *unpreventable* causes of tight muscles such as occupational, *always* stretch and hydrate often to loosen and detoxify muscles, with Shoulder Shrugs, Neck and Lower Back Stretches, etc.

*Your *body* is your best friend, take care of it, and it will take care of you!

Hmmm . . . Human Habits

OUCH illustrations and ***Ahhh*** explanations

teaches you awareness and ergonomics

with simplicity and ease,

so *Ergonomics for Proper Posture*

becomes second-nature to you . . .

Ahhh . . . Feel & Look Human Again!

Ergonomics for Proper Posture

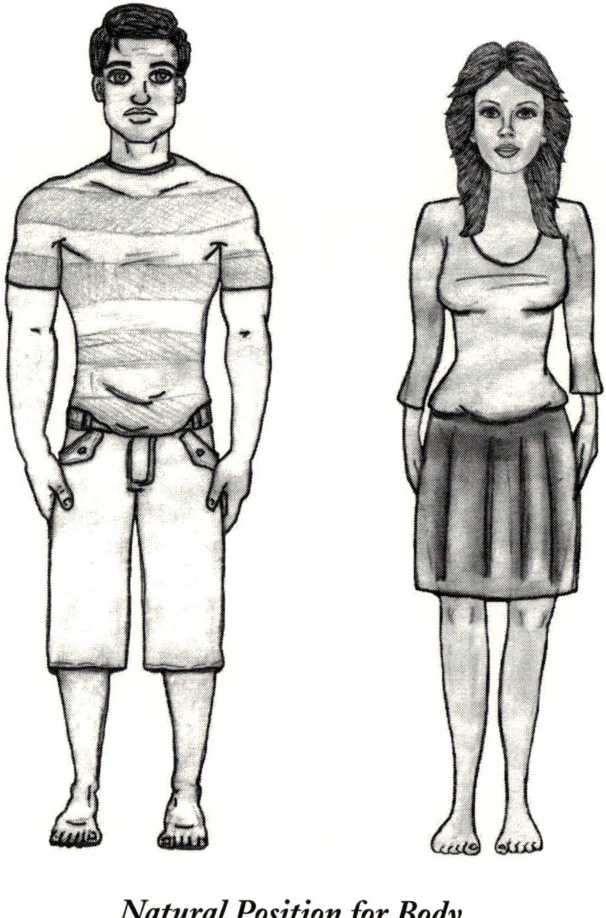

Natural Position for Body
Head straight and arms below shoulders
in stand, sit, or sleep positions

Ergonomics for Proper Posture at Work, School, Play or Rest!

Head and chin straight

Arms below shoulders

Knees, feet, and hips in alignment

Knees bent slightly, if standing

Medium support for neck, lower back, and feet

**Ergonomics* support your body *naturally*
for ease of movement and comfort.

Hmmm ... Human Habits

OUCH Back, neck, shoulders, arms,
elbows, wrists, and hands

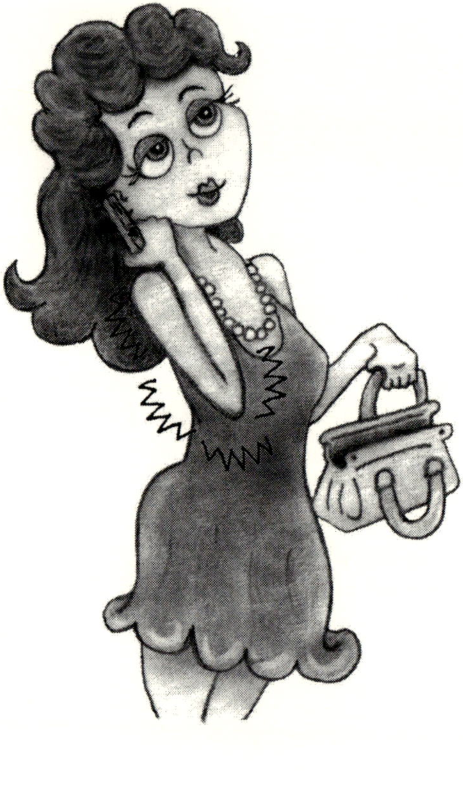

Oh Heck, my Neck ... !

Head turn or tilt, and/or shoulder up, and elbow bent

Ahhh

Problems - all *unnatural* positions, *especially* for a length of time

- turn or tilt of head
- raise shoulder up
- elbow bend – Cubitol Tunnel Syndrome (cell phone elbow)
- phones, heavy purse, briefcase, etc.
- *not* a recommendation – but *if* you must do it, switch sides *often*!

**Solutions* – ergonomics and options

- head and chin *straight*
- arms and elbows *down*
- use *hands-free* options such as a headset, ear bud, speaker phone, Bluetooth etc.
- use other *options* such as a money clip, waist or fanny pack, messenger bag, rolling briefcase, etc.

Hmmm . . . Human Habits

OUCH Back, neck, shoulders, arms, elbows, wrists, and hands

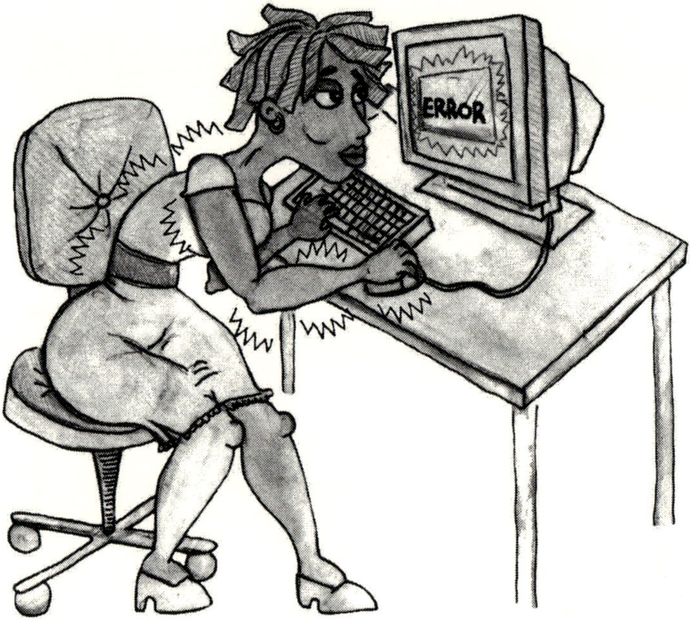

TurnHead.com!

Head turn or tilt, and no back or wrists support

Ahhh

**Problems* - all *unnatural* positions, *especially* for a length of time

- turn or tilt of head
- lack of or improper wrists support – Carpal Tunnel Syndrome
- repetitive overuse of arms and hands with mouse, etc.
- computer, TV, phone, reading materials, at conferences and seminars, etc.
- sleep habits with head turn or tilt to side, such as stomach-sleep or back

**Solutions* – ergonomics and options

- head and chin *straight,* with eyes level
- proper wrists support
- move computer, TV, etc. directly in front of you, or vice versa
- *natural* sleep positions, such as either side or back, with head *straight*

Hmmm ... Human Habits

OUCH Back, neck, shoulders, arms, elbows, wrists, and hands

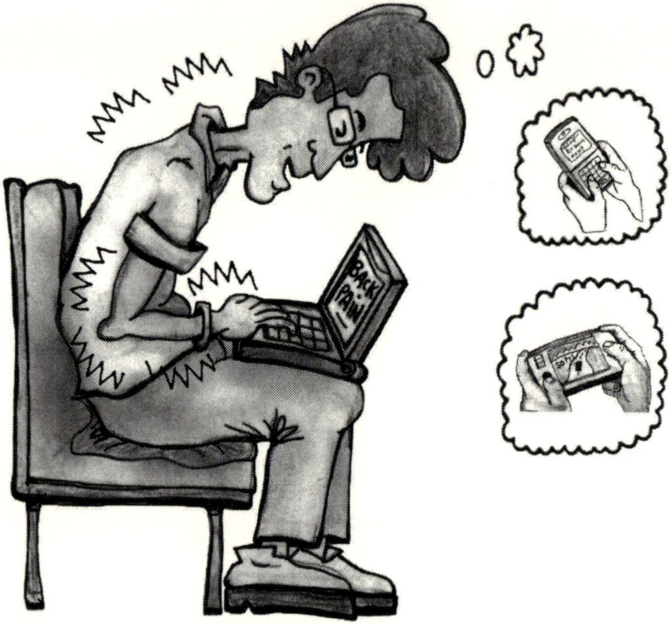

Hanging Down is a No-no!

Head down, and no back or wrists support

Ahhh

**Problems* – all *unnatural* positions, *especially* for a length of time

- head *weight* pulls muscles at neck-shoulder connection *if* up or down
- lack of or improper back support
- lack of or improper wrists support and repetitive overuse with mouse, texts, etc.
- Carpal Tunnel Syndrome (wrist)
- Thumb Tendonitis (texting)
- lack of or improper eyewear
- computer, phone, blackberry, video games, reading materials, eye glasses, etc.

**Solutions* – ergonomics and options

- head and chin *straight,* with eyes level
- proper wrists support
- prescription eyewear when reading, *if* necessary
- move computer, etc. directly in front of you, or vice versa

Hmmm ... Human Habits

OUCH Back, neck, shoulders, and elbows

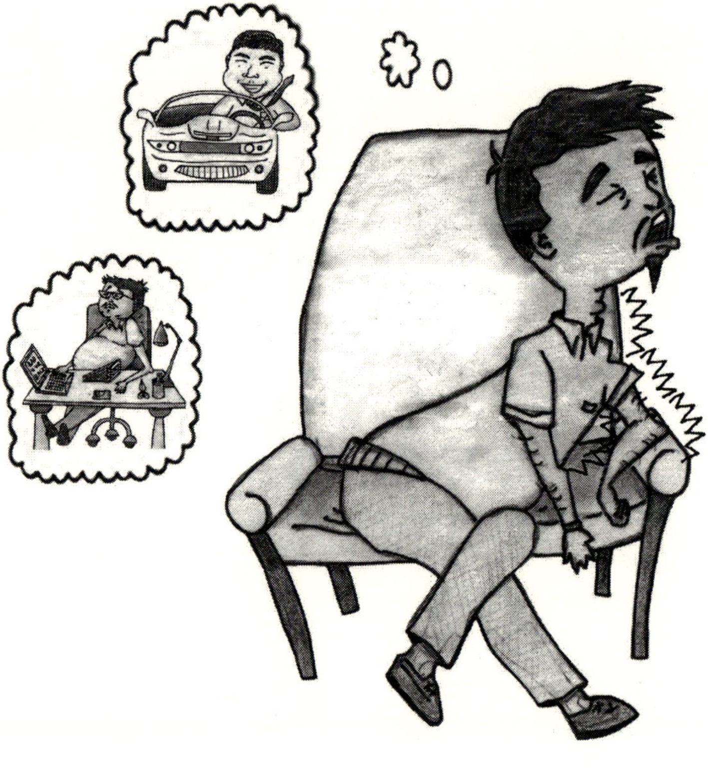

Ouch for Slouch!

Lean/slouch with no back support, and leg crosses

Ahhh

**Problems* - all *unnatural* positions, *especially* for a length of time

- lean or slouch
- lack of or improper back support
- elbow lean – Cubitol Tunnel Syndrome (cell phone elbow)
- leg crosses
- carry extra weight on *one* side, such as wallet or purse

**Solutions* – ergonomics and options

- sit *straight* with back against chair
- use proper support for back, and side if necessary
- stand *straight* with proper arch support for feet
- support elbow(s) naturally
- cross legs *only* when necessary
- use other *options* such as a money clip, waist or fanny pack, etc.

Hmmm . . . Human Habits

OUCH Lower back, legs, and feet

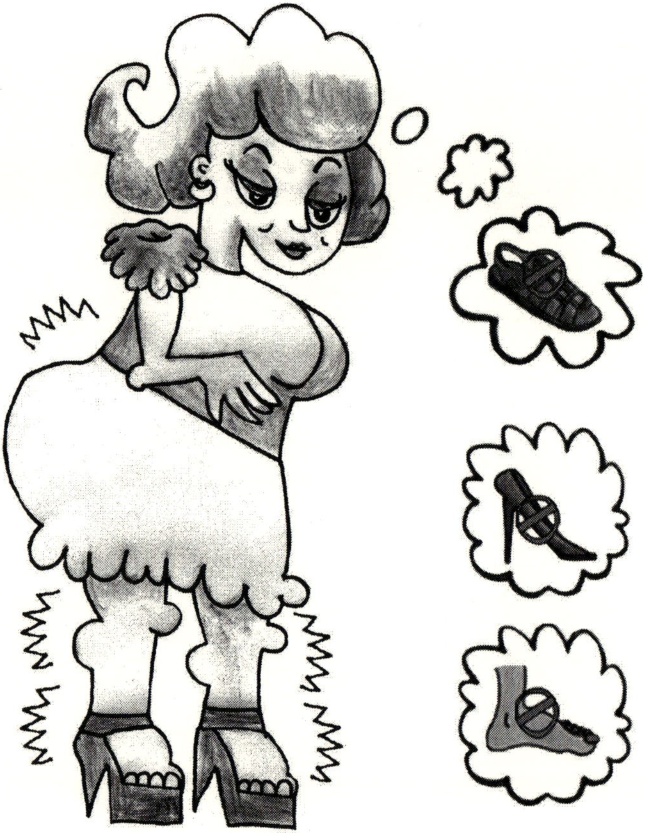

Feet Feel Funky . . . !

Improper arch support

Ahhh

**Problems* – all *unnatural* positions, *especially* for a length of time

- lack of or improper arch support
- *barefoot* – no arch support
- *flats* – usually no arch support
- *high heels* – arch on upward angle

**Solutions* – ergonomics and options

- always use proper support for *arch* of feet
- even body weight on *both* feet
- wear flat shoes *with* arch support
- barefoot or high heels *only* when necessary

Hmmm … Human Habits

OUCH Upper/lower back, neck, and shoulders

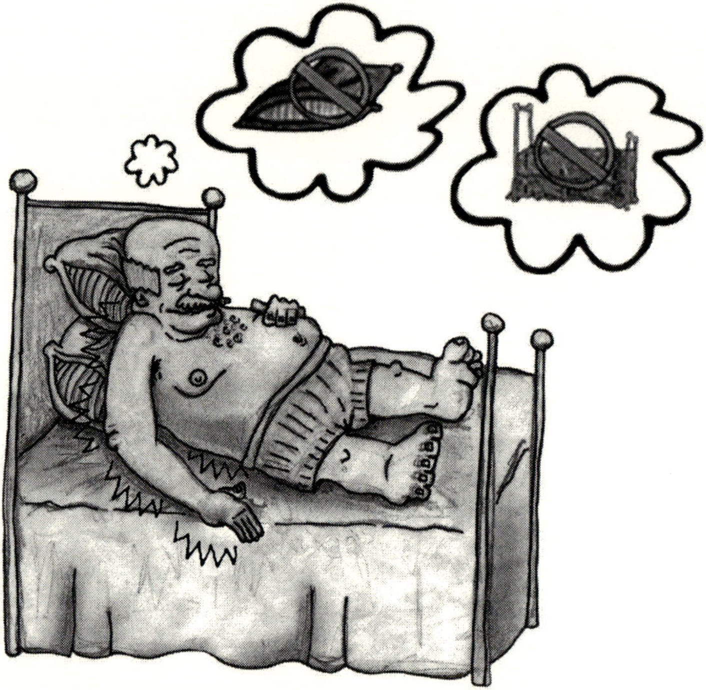

Sleepless in Slumber!

No pillow or flat pillow – too low

Too many pillows – too high

Ahhh

**Problems* – all *unnatural* positions, *especially* for a length of time

- lack of or improper neck support
- *no* pillow – tilts chin *up*
- *flat* pillow – tilts chin *up*
- *firm* or *too many* pillows – tilts chin *down*
- chin *up* or *down* causes tight muscles, *especially* at the neck-shoulder connection

**Solutions* – ergonomics and options

- *medium* neck support, with chin *straight*
- use *medium* support for lower back -
  under knees for back sleepers, and *between* knees for side sleepers
- neck support with a *medium* pillow opens airway naturally to help *prevent* snoring and restlessness

**break* habit - since we are *Creatures of Habit, remove* flat and/or extra pillow(s) from bed and surroundings since we are *Creatures of Habit*

- see *Physician* and/or *Healthcare Practitioner* if too many pillows are necessary due to sinus congestion, heartburn, acid reflux, asthma, etc.

Hmmm . . . Human Habits

OUCH Lower/upper back, neck, shoulders, arm(s), and leg(s)

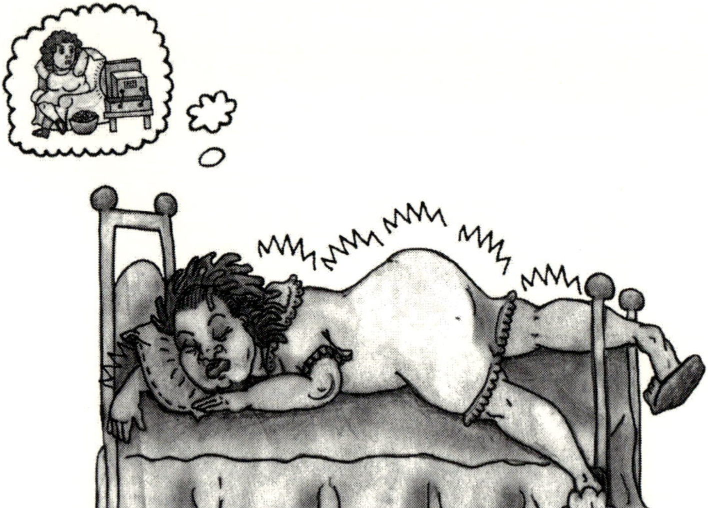

Don't do the Twist and Turn!

Stomach-sleeping with head turn and arm(s) above shoulder(s)

Ahhh

******Problems* – an *unnatural* sleep position, *especially* for a length of time

- head turn to side and arms(s) up above shoulder(s) or outward

******imagine* these *unnatural* position if you *stand* or *sit* with your head turned to *one* side and arm(s) above shoulder(s)

******Solutions* – ergonomics and options

- sleep in *natural* positions - back or either side
- *back* or *side* sleep positions with proper neck support opens airway naturally to help *prevent* snoring and restlessness
- *back sleepers* – keep head *straight* to *prevent* tight back, neck, and shoulders, *especially* on one side
- *side sleepers* – sleep on the side of your head and *not* your face to *prevent* premature wrinkles
- once your head *weight* is on pillow with *either* side or back sleep, keep chin *staight*

* *break* habit with a *firm* pillow or body *pillow*

- *back sleepers* - put pillow on *one* or *both* sides, and arms *down* by sides or on stomach
- *side sleepers* – put pillow in *front* of stomach, and arms *down* and around pillow

Hmmm ... Human Habits

OUCH Premature wrinkles to face

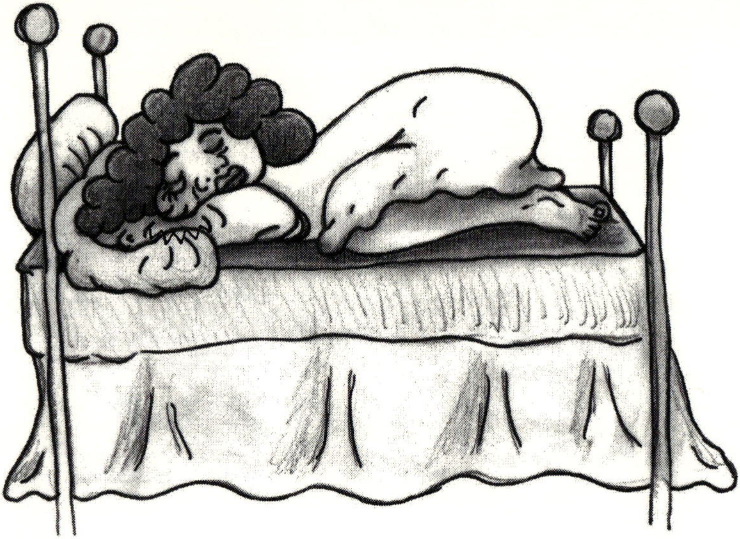

Wrinkles–Oh, No!

Stomach-sleeping wrinkles skin, *especially* on one side

Ahhh

******Problems* – all *unnatural* positions, *especially* for a length of time

- premature wrinkles on *one* side of face
- sleep habits such as stomach sleepers – skin *pulls* on side of face on pillow
- support of face in hand(s) – skin *pulls* on side of face in hand(s)

******Solutions* – ergonomics and options

- sleep in *natural* positions - back or either side
- *side sleepers* - sleep on the side of your head and *not* your face to *prevent* premature facial wrinkles
- do *not* support your forehead, cheeks, and/or chin in your hands

Hmmm . . . Human Habits

OUCH Jaw, upper back, neck, shoulders, arms, and hands

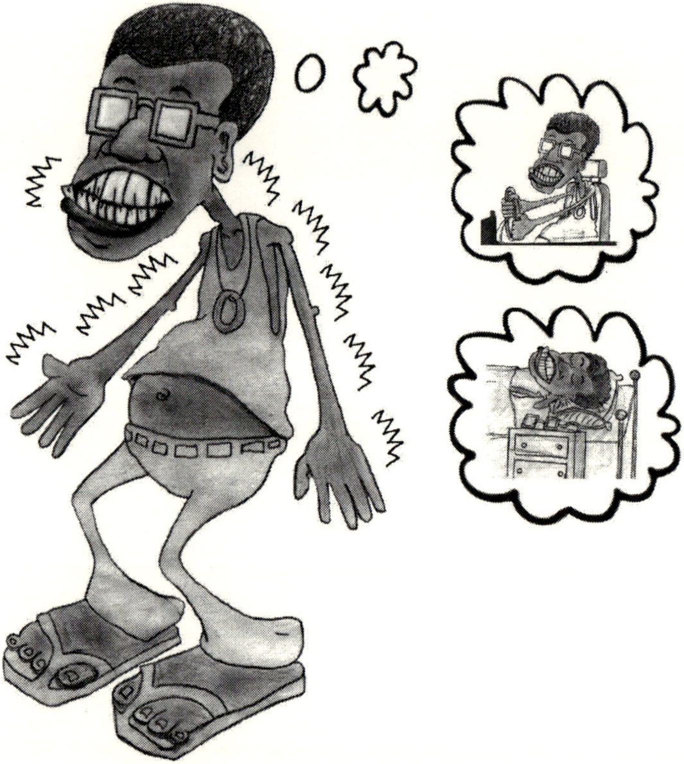

Pain in the Face . . . !

Clench and/or grind jaw and teeth at work, school, play, or rest

Ahhh

**Problems* – all *unnatural* positions, *especially* for a length of time

- clench and/or grind of jaw and teeth
- *constant* clench and grind causes tight muscles, potential pinch of nerves, and may trigger headaches
- *constant* grind of teeth causes tooth and gum problems
- clench and/or grind is usually done *both* day and night

**constant* jaw movement is *unnatural,* imagine doing the *chew* movement for a length of time

**Solutions* – ergonomics and options

- awareness, correction, and stretches

* *break* habit of clench/grind *during the day*

- be *aware* of your clench/grind
- mentally *and* verbally tell yourself *no*
- breathe *slowly* and *deeply* as you *stretch* your jaw with a big yawn
- hold *open yawn* for 5–10 seconds
- release and repeat often
- *stretch* to *release* tight back, neck, and shoulders with Shoulder Shrugs and Neck stretches
- see *Dentist* – use mouth guard to protect teeth and gums *while you sleep*

Hmmm . . . Human Habits

OUCH Lower back, legs, feet, and joints

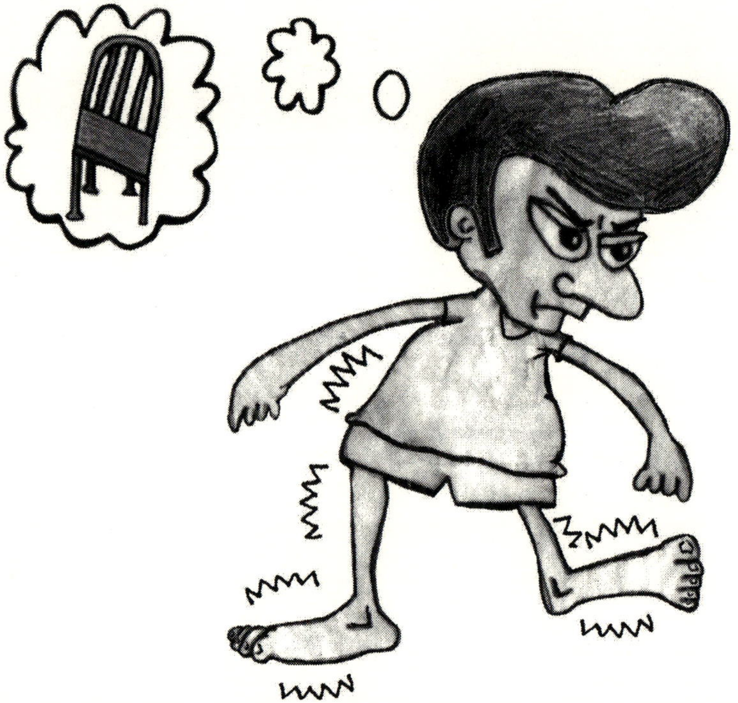

Hobbling Hurts!

One leg shorter than the other

Ahhh

**Problems* – an *unnatural* position, *especially* for a length of time

- *one* leg shorter than the other
- hips *uneven* due to different leg lengths
- usually your arms and legs are ¼ inch or less shorter than the other, and often it is not a problem
- *more* than ¼ inch causes tight muscles and/or joint problems
- difference is due to injury, surgery, illness and/or genetics
- sleep habits with arm(s) above shoulder(s)

**Solutions* – ergonomics and options

- *even* length of legs
- wear an insole in the shoe of your shorter leg *only*
- orthotics
- barefoot *only* when necessary
- *natural* sleep positions of back or side, with arms down *below* shoulders
- see *Physician, Podiatrist,* and/or *Healthcare Practitioner*, if necessary

Hmmm . . . Human Habits

OUCH Back, neck, shoulders, arms, legs, hands, and feet

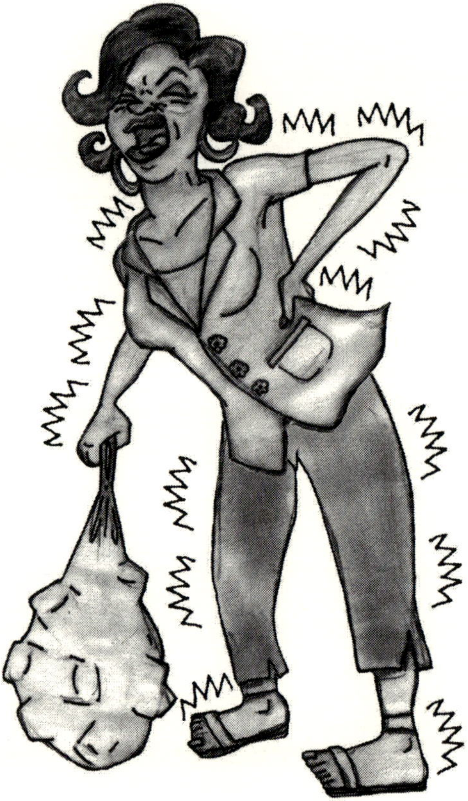

Bad Back Attack!

Misalignment of spine

Ahhh

**Problems* – all *unnatural* positions, *especially* for a length of time

- misalignment of spine
- improper lifting
- imbalance of weight
- injury, surgery, illness and/or genetics
- inflammation and tight muscles
- headaches, nerve pain and/or loss of sensation in limbs

**Solutions* – ergonomics and options

- *always* align and support body naturally
- *always* bend with your knees *first* and *not* at your waist
- *always* balance weight *before* lifting

*naturally realign with a *Rocking Stretch*

- lie on your *side* with your feet, ankles and knees in alignment, and arms outstretched, with hands together
- *slowly* and *gently* rock *side to side* –
- *begin* with your feet and ankles, then hips and lower back, next with upper back, neck, and shoulders, then arms and hands, and lastly your head
- do *rocking* movements for a *few* minutes until you feel a *comfortable* release of muscles overall
- repeat on *opposite* side, and do stretch often
- see *Physician, Chiropractor,* and/or *Healthcare Practitioner*, if necessary

Hmmm… Human Habits!

OUCH Back, neck shoulders, arms, and legs

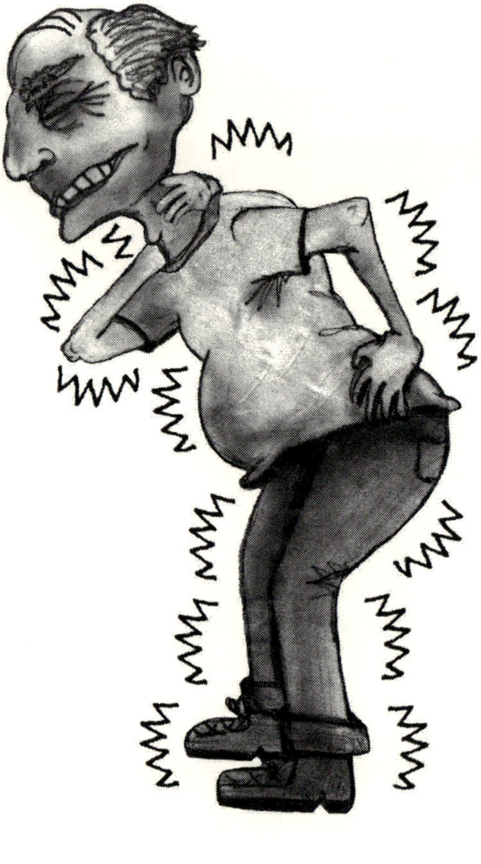

Poor Posture Pain!

Overall tight muscles

Ahhh

**Problems* – all *unnatural* positions, *especially* for a length of time

- *overall* poor posture
- lack of or improper support
- lack of flexibility
- stiffness

*Solutions – ergonomics and options

- *always* use proper posture at *work, school, play or rest*

*naturally realign with a *Squat Stretch*

- *gently* bend your knees and lower your body to a *squat* position
- hold for 5–10 seconds, then *slowly* stand up
- repeat often
- for your *saftey*, hold onto a *stationary* object when doing stretch, if necessary

Body Care Solutions

A healthy and vibrant *body* begins with your daily basics, such as a nutrient-rich diet, water, plenty of exercise and sleep, and a sunscreen.

Slow and deep *wellness breaths* soothe and calm from *within* to change how you feel and look *naturally* for immediate stress release, so you feel more peaceful.

Stretch and *exercise* often as *movement* is nutrition for your *body,* same as air, food, and water.

Ergonomics support you *naturally* and help prevent a slumping posture, *especially* with *medium* support for your neck, lower back and arch of feet.

Self massages relax and detoxify, while *natural remedies* promote healing and prevention of tight muscles and inflammation, as proper *nutrition* and *antioxidants* revitalize and protect your body for optimal health.

Stretches to Relax or Awaken

*For all stretches, always breathe *slowly* and *deeply* as you *gently* stretch to your *comfort* level *only*!

Breathe as you *raise* your arms above your shoulders and stretch your upper body and fingers, and then your lower body and toes, until you feel a *comfortable* pull overall, then release and *exhale* as you lower your arms, and repeat often.

Shoulder Shrug Stretches

*Always do stretch in a *circular* motion.

Breathe as you *raise* your shoulders up toward your ears, and *roll* your shoulders *backward* as you *squeeze* your scapulas together until you feel a *comfortable* pull, then release and *exhale* as you *roll* your shoulders *downward*, and repeat often.

Breathe as you *raise* your shoulders up toward your ears, and *roll* your shoulders *forward* as you gently *squeeze* your pectorals together until you feel a *comfortable* pull, then release and *exhale* as you *roll* your shoulders *downward*, and repeat often.

Lower Back Stretches

*Always do in a *slow* motion.

Breathe as you lean forward, and *lower* your upper body until you feel a *comfortable* pull, then release and *exhale* as you slowly raise upward, and repeat often.

Breathe as you *raise* your arms *upward* you feel a *comfortable* pull, then release and *exhale* as you slowly *lower* your arms, and repeat often.

Neck Stretches

*Always do stretch in a *slow* motion.

Breathe as you *turn* your head to *one* side until you feel a *comfortable* pull, then release and *exhale* as you return your head to *center*, and repeat with opposite side, and do stretch often.

Breathe as you *lower* your head *forward* until you feel a *comfortable* pull, then release and *exhale* as you return your head to *center*, and repeat often.

Breathe as you *lower* your head *backward* until you feel a *comfortable* pull, then release and *exhale* as you return your head to *center*, and repeat often.

Ergonomic Body Positions

For *natural* support and comfort while you *sit, stand,* or *sleep*

- *Sit*
  - » rest your buttocks *against* the back of your chair to naturally support your upper and lower back
  - » *align* your knees and feet even with your hips
  - » use *lumbar* support for your lower back, *if* necessary
- *Stand*
  - » roll your shoulders *backward* and tuck your stomach *inward*
  - » use proper *arch* support for your feet
- *Sleep*
  - » *natural* sleep positions, back or either side, with *medium* support under your neck
  - » support *lower back* -
back sleepers - *under* your knees
side sleepers - *between* your knees

Self-Massage with Acupressure

Acupressure stimulates specific points for your vital energy, *Qi*, to flow freely through your body as it shifts excess energy away from congestion.

For example, the *Union Valley Point*, located between your thumb and index finger, relaxes tight muscles and relieves headaches.

* Breathe as you gently press *above* and *below* point with a *comfortable* pressure using your opposite hand, and hold for *20–30* seconds, then release and repeat on *opposite* hand, and massage often.

Self-Massage with a Tennis Ball

A *foot* massage relaxes tight muscles, e*specially* heel and arch pain, and stimulates *reflexology* points to detoxify your entire body.

Relax your feet with a soak or shower *before* massage for less sensitivity and deeper penetration.

* Breathe as you *gently* roll the tennis ball under your foot using your body weight with a *comfortable* pressure, and hold for a *few* seconds on *sensitive* areas, then release and repeat on *opposite* foot, and stretch often.

*For your safety *during* massage, place the tennis ball on a *non-skid* surface and hold onto a *stationary* object.

Natural Remedies for a Healthy Body

Tight Muscles and Inflammation

- heal and prevent with *Ergonomics for Proper Posture*
- apply *heat* to relax tight muscles and increase circulation
- apply *cold* to reduce swelling and decrease circulation
- apply cold and moist heat *alternately* for 15 minutes every hour

De-stress

- relax with a hot shower or bath *before* bed
- renew with plenty of sleep

Food Pyramid

- whole grains
- dark green and orange vegetables
- dry beans and peas
- fresh, frozen, canned or dry fruit (less fruit juices)
- low fat or fat-free dairy, or lactose-free

- low fat or lean meats, poultry or fish (bake, broil or grill)
- nuts and seeds
- healthy sugars

Water

- essential for a healthy body
- hydrate often and daily

Antioxidants

- spices, *especially* curcumin or tumeric, and cinnamon
- dark chocolate and cocoa – release *endorphins* also

Detoxify

- teas, *especially* green and black
- apple cider vinegar

* Your *lifespan* is *20% genes, and 80% lifestyle*!

Ergonomics for Proper Posture with *awareness* will help you -

Ahhh... Feel & Look Human Again!

Skin Care for a Natural Appearance

- Stress is not the *only* cause of your skin problems!
- Your premature facial wrinkles and blemishes are the *symptoms* and not the problem!
- The problem is the *root cause(s)* of your skin concerns!

Often the *root causes* of your premature facial wrinkles and blemishes are just a lack of or improper skin care and sleep habits.

Surprisingly, these problems are easily *preventable* with some simple lifestyle changes, such as a basic *skin care recipe* and *natural* sleep positions.

The answer is not to treat your symptoms *only*, as it usually just masks the problem, may be ineffective, and cause possible side effects.

The *real* answer is to always treat the *root cause(s)* of your skin problems for relief and results.

Overall your premature facial wrinkles and skin problems are *unhealthy* as they cause stress and discomfort, just to name a few!

What are *you* doing to create your symptoms?

Usually, it is your *often-known or unknown* lifestyle habits, *especially* for a length of time at *work*, *school*, *play* or *rest*!

....

Since your premature facial wrinkles are usually more on *one* side of your face, most often it is due to *sleep* habits such as being on your stomach with your face on the pillow, as it *pulls* your skin.

Your blemishes are usually more on *one* area of your face and most often due to *lifestyle* habits such as poor diet, hormones, and unclean hand(s) or items on skin.

Lack of or wrong skin care products for your *specific* skin type cause skin problems for *all* skin types.

Stress will intensify your skin problems, but it is *not* the *root cause* alone!

**If* it were *only* stress, you would see the *same* premature facial wrinkles and blemishes *all* over your face, and not *more* in just one or two areas.

Some *problem* areas and usual *root causes* due to improper skin care and sleep habits, *especially* for a length of time

- *Forehead*
    - » hair, such as bangs on skin
    - » sleep habits *pulls* skin
    - » stress lines

- *Eyes*
    - » lack of or improper skin care above *and* below eyes
    - » lack of or improper eyewear causes squints
    - » sleep habits or face in hand(s) *pulls* skin

- *Cheeks*
    - » daily diet of food and drink
    - » sleep habits or cheek(s) in hand(s) *pulls* skin
    - » unclean hands or items on skin, such as phone

- *Lips*
    - » lack of or improper skim care above *and* below lips
    - » pucker of lips

- *Chin*
  - » hormonal, especially premenstrual
  - » sleep habits or chin in hand(s) *pulls* skin
  - » unclean hands or items on skin, such as phone

- *Neck, Décollete, and Ears*
  - » lack of or improper skin care to all areas

*Any *untouched* skin causes skin problems eventually!

....

Although use of a few skin care products gives you *temporary* results, it is simply *not* enough to undue the *many* hours of lack of or improper skin care and sleep habits!

Once you go back to your *often-known or unknown* lifestyle habits, you create the *same* premature facial wrinkles and skin problems *sooner* rather than later!

Some lifestyle changes, such as *Skin Care for a Natural Appearance,* help you be part of the solution and…

Ahhh… Feel & Look Human Again!

Some *preventable* and *unpreventable* usual *root causes* of skin problems, *especially* for a length of time

- lack of or improper skin care
- lack of sunscreen
- poor diet and posture
- dehydration and deficiency
- hormonal imbalance
- overabundance of stress of fatigue
- lack of sleep and exercise
- sleep habits such as stomach-sleeping
- congestion of toxins and lack of oxygen
- support of face in hand(s)
- injury or surgery
- illness or genetics
- pregnancy
- elderly and natural aging
- occupational

- negative emotions –
- anger and resentment, anxiety, fear, and grief

*Negative emotions prematurely age your skin

The *good* news is that your *preventable* and *unpreventable* premature facial wrinkles and skin problems can lessen or even disappear once you stop the *root cause(s)*!

For *unpreventable* skin problems, *always* do a daily *skin care recipe* and hydrate to replenish and detoxify your skin!

* Your *skin* is your best friend, take care of it, and it will take care of you!

Hmmm ... Skin Care

Skin Care illustrations and explanations with *recipe*

teaches you awareness and proper skin

care with simplicity and ease,

so *Skin Care for a Natural Appearance*

becomes second-nature to you ...

Ahhh ... Feel & Look Human Again!

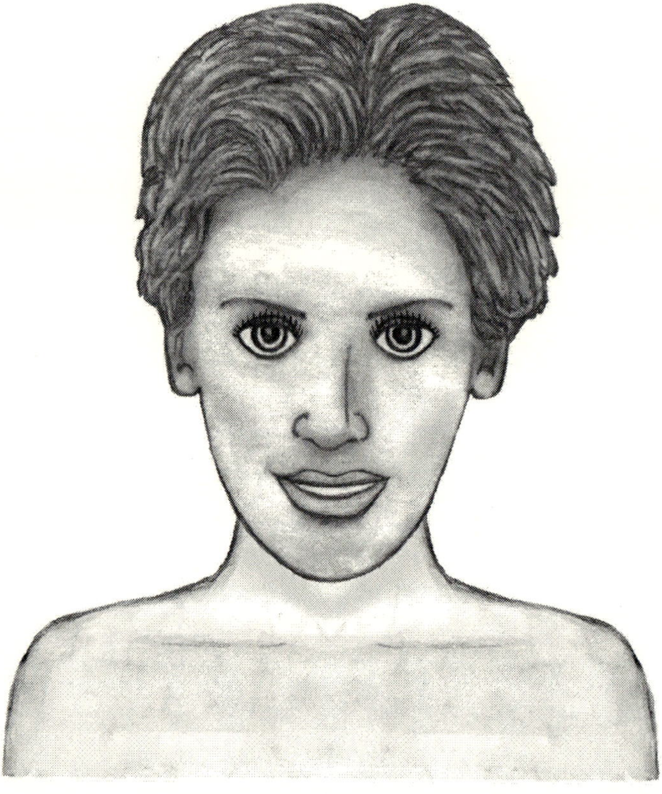

Ladies, you look like Sisters!

Natural and healthy youthful appearance

Hmmm ... Skin Care for Men

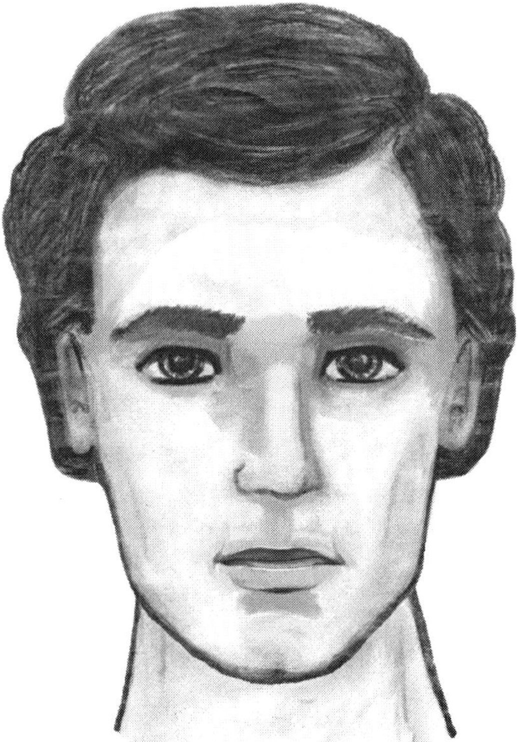

Is it Dad or Son?

Natural and healthy youthful appearance

Skin Care Recipe

Skin care is just like your favorite dish or dessert *recipe!*

Preparation with *all* of the ingredients creates awesome results, but *if* you miss one or two, there is a problem?

S*ame* is true for your skin!

A daily *skin care recipe* helps to minimize, correct and prevent premature facial wrinkles and skin problems such as congestion, dehydration, enlarged pores, and uneven skin tone, just to name a few!

Always apply skin care products to your face, neck, décolleté, ears, and head if bald or shaven, with *upward* strokes and *light* fingertip pressure.

*Any *untouched* skin shows premature facial wrinkles and skin problems *sooner* rather than later.

....

Always use skin care products for your skin type *only* to prevent skin problems and to encourage your natural anti-aging defenses.

- *Sensitive* skin products are gentle to soothe and calm, and to prevent reactions
- *Dry* skin products are creamy and rich to hydrate and nourish skin
- *Oily* skin products are light to deep cleanse and purify skin
- *Normal-combination* skin products are ideal for skin that is not overly dry or oily
- *Anti-aging* skin products are best to correct and prevent wrinkles, loss of elasticity, etc.

**Dry* skin products cause congestion on *oily* skin since texture is too heavy
**Oily* skin products cause dehydration on *dry* skin since they purify

**Emulsify* your skin care products with a small amount of water for a *lighter* application, if necessary.

....

A daily *skin care recipe*, morning *and* night, is essential for the overall health and appearance of your skin.

- *Morning Recipe*
  - » cleanser, toner, serum(s), eye cream, moisturizer, sunscreen, and lip care

- *Night Recipe*
  - » cleanser, exfoliant, toner, serum(s), eye cream, moisturizer, and lip care

Skin Care Recipe

- *Cleansers*
  - » remove impurities to refresh appearance
  - » apply *daily* in a *circular* motion for a smooth application

- *Exfoliants and Peels*
  - » refine to remove dead skin and unclog pores
  - » apply *daily* on cleansed skin for renewal and vibrancy

- *Toners*
  - » remove residue
  - » balance PH levels to give skin a natural healthy glow
  - » spray on *cleansed* skin for refreshment
  - » apply *daily* for best results

- *Serums*
  - » prevents premature aging and skin problems for all skin types, ethnicities, and ages
  - » apply a few drops with *light* fingertip pressure
  - » apply *daily* for best results

**Sensitive* skin to soothe, calm and nourish
**Oily* skin to heal, repair and prevent
**Dry* skin to hydrate, replenish and plump
**Anti-age* to lighten, tone and firm

- *Eye Makeup Remover*
  - » cleanse and protect eye areas
  - » apply *gently* for removal

- *Eye Exfoliants*
  - » minimize fine lines and crow's feet for a more youthful appearance
  - » apply *weekly* for best results

- *Eye Masks*
    - » calm and hydrate to increase smoothness and elasticity
    - » apply *weekly* for best results

- *Eye Creams, Gels and Balms*
    - » refresh and firm to reduce puffiness and dark circles
    - » apply *daily* to contour areas below *and* above eyes with a *gentle* tap motion

- *Moisturizers*
    - » hydrate, clarify and firm for a healthy and youthful appearance
    - » apply *daily* with gentle *upward* strokes morning and night

- *Sunscreen*
    - » minimize the harmful effects of the sun
    - » helps protect the youth and elasticity of your skin
    - » apply *daily*, and use often if outdoors

- *Lip Exfoliants*
    - » remove dryness and refine fine vertical lip lines for smoothness
    - » apply *weekly* for best results

- *Lip Masks*
  - » soothe and hydrate to increase smoothness and suppleness
  - » apply *weekly* for best results

- *Lip Balms*
  - » hydrate and plump lips for a more youthful appearance
  - » apply *daily* to lips and contour areas above *and* below to prevent vertical lip lines, *especially* before bed

- *Masks*
  - » encourage a deeper penetration to calm, hydrate, heal, nurture, and increase elasticity
  - » apply *weekly* for best results

- *Blemish Control*
  - » heal and cover for a healthy appearance
  - » apply on blemishes, *especially* before bed

Expiration Dates

Skin *reactions* are often due to an allergy, sensitivity, contamination, or expiration of products.

Just like groceries, your skin care products *only* last so long.

Once *open*, they can last up to two years in a jar and three years in a pump. Sunscreen lasts one year and often has an expiration date on it.

Always write down the date when you open you skin care products.

Old skin care products can spoil and irritate your skin, being unsafe to use and ineffective also.

This *is* true regardless of pharmaceutical, high-end, or even organic products.

Dispose of skin care products *if* you notice a change in smell or consistency, or *if* you have a reaction or infection seek medical attention, *if* necessary.

*What you put on your skin *is* almost as important as what you eat and drink!

Skin Care Solutions

Healthy and radiant *skin* begins with your daily basics such as a nutrient-rich diet, water, plenty of exercise and sleep, and a sunscreen.

Slow and deep *beauty breaths* detoxify your skin from *within* to change how you look and feel naturally for immediate stress release, so you look more youthful.

Stretch and *exercise* often as *movement* is nutrition for your *skin*, the same as air, food and water.

Ergonomics support you *naturally* and help prevent premature facial wrinkles, *especially* with *natural* sleep positions such as your back or either side.

Facial massages relax and detoxify, while *natural remedies* promote healing and prevention of blemishes and premature aging, as proper *nutrition and antioxidants* revitalize and protect your skin for optimal health.

Facial Massage

A f*acial massage* nourishes your *skin* with fresh oxygen and circulation as it cleanses from *within* to improve elasticity and reduce puffiness for a more youthful appearance *naturally*.

Do your *Skin Care Recipe*, then start massage –

- emulsify moisturizer using *moist* fingertips
- always use *light* fingertip pressure with slow *horizontal* strokes
- begin your facial massage from the *top* and *center* of your face, *outward* to your hairline and ears, being *especially* gentle around eye areas
- *gently* apply *light* pressure and *slowly* glide across your face
    - » breathe slowly and deeply
    - » *begin* massage with the top and center of your forehead to your hairline
    - » then *gently* press under your eyebrows to your temples
    - » under your eyes to your temples
    - » down your nose and across your cheeks to your ears
    - » under your nose and across your cheeks to your jaw line
    - » across your chin to your jaw line
    - » follow your jaw line to your ears
    - » *gently* massage ears

*Repeat *massage* often to relax and renew for a natural and healthy appearance.

Natural Remedies for Healthy Skin

Congestion and Blemishes

- clarify and purify daily with *Skin Care Recipe*
- wash your hands *before* cleansing your face
- avoid touching your face with unclean hands
- cleanse your phone daily since it touches your ear, cheeks and chin when in use
- apply blemish control as *picking* may leave marks or scars

*For *extractions*, always use *light* fingertip pressure and apply toner afterwards

*For acne or unusual marks, growths, etc. – see your *Dermatologist*

Dehydration and Premature Aging

- replenish and renew daily with *Skin Care Recipe*
- hydrate frequently
- apply a sunscreen and use often *if* outdoors

*For rosacea, hyper-pigmentation, etc. – see your *Dermatologist*

De-stress

- relax with a hot shower or bath *before* bed
- renew with plenty of sleep

Food Pyramid

- whole grains
- dark green and orange vegetables
- dry beans and peas
- fresh, frozen, canned or dried fruit (less fruit juices)
- low fat or fat-free dairy, lactose-free
- low fat or lean meats, poultry or fish (bake, broil or grill)
- nuts and seeds
- healthy sugars

Water

- essential for healthy skin
- hydrate often daily

Antioxidants

- spices, *especially* curcumin or tumeric, and cinnamon
- dark chocolate and cocoa – release *endorphins* also

Detoxify

- teas, *especially* green and black
- apple cider vinegar

* Your *skinspan* is 20% genes, and *80% lifestyle*!

Skin Care for a Natural Appearance with *Recipe* will help you -

Ahhh... Feel & Look Human Again!